VEGETARIAN KIDNEY DISEASE COOKBOOK

Delicious and Nutritious Recipes to Help Manage Kidney Disease

Dr Lily Morgan

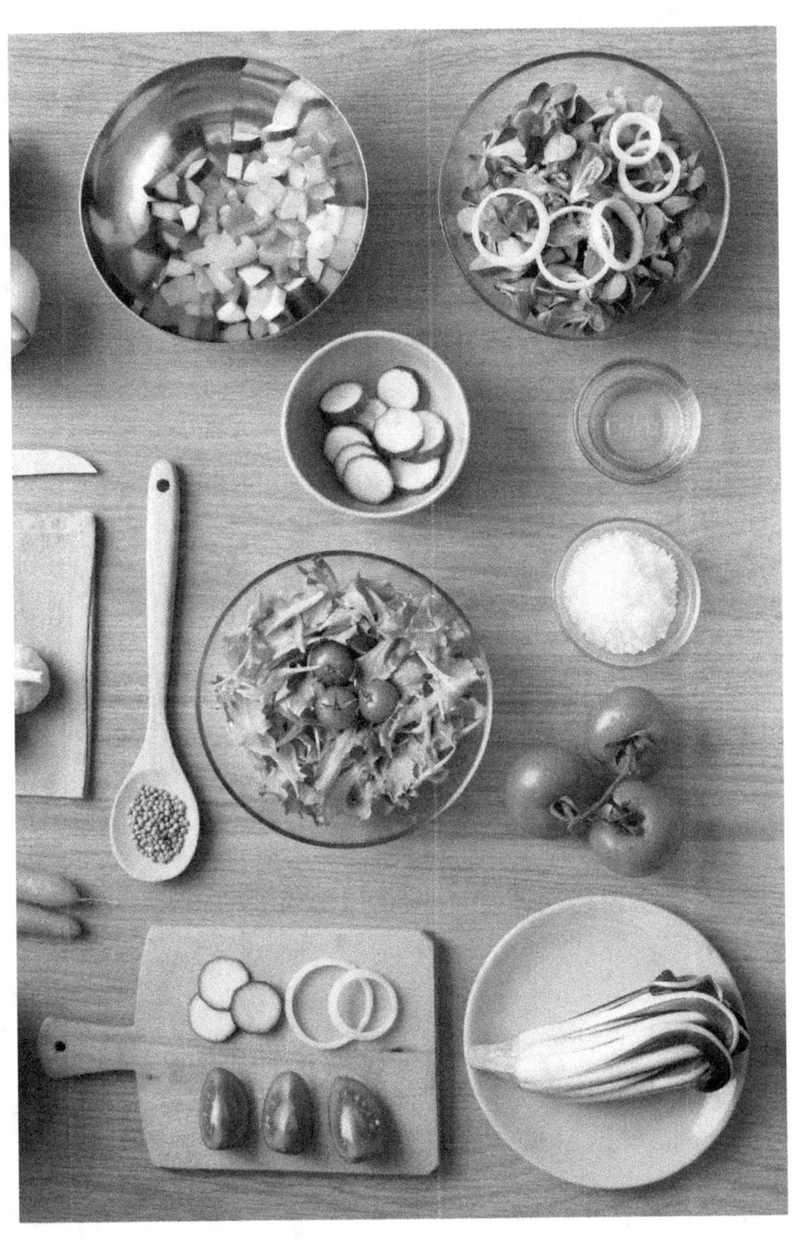

TABLE OF CONTENTS

Chapter 3: Lunch Recipes...................................... 36

Chapter 6: Desserts 97

INTRODUCTION

K idney disease is a complex and often silent condition that affects millions of people worldwide. It's crucial to comprehend how this ailment interacts with your diet to make informed choices for your health.

Your kidneys play a pivotal role in maintaining overall health. They act as natural filters, eliminating waste and excess fluids from your blood, regulating electrolyte levels, and producing hormones that control blood pressure. When kidney function deteriorates, these functions become compromised.

Diet is a critical component in managing kidney disease. By understanding the relationship between kidney health and nutrition, you can take proactive steps to slow the progression of the disease and improve your quality of life. Here are key points to consider:

1. **Sodium Control:** High sodium intake can raise blood pressure and lead to fluid retention. Reducing salt in your diet is vital for kidney health.

2. **Protein Moderation:** Protein breakdown creates waste products that the kidneys must filter. Adjusting your protein intake to match your kidney function is essential.

3. **Fluid Management:** Kidneys struggling with disease may have difficulty regulating fluid levels. Monitoring your fluid intake is crucial to avoid dehydration or excessive fluid retention.

4. **Phosphorus and Potassium Awareness**: Elevated levels of these minerals can harm your bones and heart. Managing foods rich in phosphorus and potassium is essential.

Tips for Managing Kidney Disease with a Vegetarian Diet:

Switching to a vegetarian diet can be an excellent choice for kidney disease management, as plant-based foods are often lower in protein and provide a variety of nutrients beneficial for kidney health. Here are some tips for navigating a vegetarian diet with kidney disease:

1. **Balanced Protein:** Incorporate high-quality plant protein sources like legumes, tofu, and tempeh while moderating your intake.

2. **Limit High-Potassium Foods:** Be mindful of potassium-rich foods like bananas, oranges, and potatoes. Cooking methods like soaking and boiling can reduce potassium content.

3. **Control Phosphorus:** Keep track of phosphorus in dairy alternatives and whole grains. Choose lower phosphorus options when possible.

4. **Monitor Fluids:** Pay attention to your fluid intake, as some vegetarian foods like soups and stews can be high in liquids.

5. **Work with a Dietitian:** Consult a registered dietitian who specializes in kidney disease and vegetarian diets. They can provide personalized guidance and meal plans tailored to your needs.

Remember, managing kidney disease with a vegetarian diet requires a thoughtful and individualized approach. Regular monitoring and collaboration with healthcare professionals are key to your long-term well-being.

Chapter 1: 30-Day Meal Plan

Week 1:

Day 1:

- Breakfast: Nutrient-Packed Smoothie Bowl
- Lunch: Chickpea and Avocado Salad
- Dinner: Mushroom and Spinach Stuffed Shells
- Snacks: Guacamole and Veggie Sticks
- Dessert: Berry and Banana Ice Cream

Day 2:

- Breakfast: Spinach and Mushroom Omelette
- Lunch: Lentil Soup with Spinach
- Dinner: Vegan Chili
- Snacks: Roasted Red Pepper Hummus
- Dessert: Chocolate Avocado Mousse

Day 3:

- Breakfast: Quinoa Breakfast Bowl
- Lunch: Caprese Quinoa Salad
- Dinner: Ratatouille

- Snacks: Edamame with Sea Salt
- Dessert: Vegan Rice Pudding

Day 4:

- Breakfast: Blueberry Chia Pudding
- Lunch: Roasted Veggie Wrap
- Dinner: Lemon Herb Baked Tofu
- Snacks: Cucumber and Tomato Bruschetta
- Dessert: Apple Cinnamon Crisp

Day 5:

- Breakfast: Vegetable Breakfast Burrito
- Lunch: Black Bean and Corn Salad
- Dinner: Spinach and Ricotta Cannelloni
- Snacks: Baked Sweet Potato Fries
- Dessert: Chia Seed Pudding with Berries

Day 6:

- Breakfast: Oatmeal with Fresh Berries
- Lunch: Spinach and Mushroom Quesadilla
- Dinner: Sweet Potato and Lentil Curry
- Snacks: Stuffed Mushrooms

- Dessert: Baked Pears with Cinnamon

Day 7:

- Breakfast: Greek Yogurt Parfait
- Lunch: Mediterranean Farro Salad
- Dinner: Butternut Squash Risotto
- Snacks: Spinach and Artichoke Dip
- Dessert: Vegan Chocolate Chip Cookies

Week 2

Day 8:

- Breakfast: Avocado Toast with Poached Egg
- Lunch: Sweet Potato and Black Bean Bowl
- Dinner: Portobello Mushroom Steaks
- Snacks: Mixed Nuts and Dried Fruit
- Dessert: Blueberry Oat Bars

Day 9:

- Breakfast: Banana Walnut Pancakes
- Lunch: Tofu Stir-Fry
- Dinner: Black Bean Enchiladas
- Snacks: Caprese Skewers

- Dessert: Coconut Mango Sorbet

Day 10:

- Breakfast: Tofu Scramble
- Lunch: Greek Salad with Tzatziki Dressing
- Dinner: Thai Vegetable Green Curry
- Snacks: Vegan Spring Rolls with Peanut Sauce
- Dessert: Chocolate Covered Strawberries

Day 11:

- Breakfast: Breakfast Quiche
- Lunch: Quinoa and Vegetable Stuffed Peppers
- Dinner: Eggplant Rollatini
- Snacks: Deviled Eggs (Vegan)
- Dessert: Pumpkin Pie Smoothie

Day 12:

- Breakfast: Coconut Mango Rice Pudding
- Lunch: Tomato Basil Soup
- Dinner: Quinoa Stuffed Acorn Squash
- Snacks: Spicy Chickpea Snack
- Dessert: Almond Joy Energy Bites

Day 13:

- Breakfast: Sweet Potato Hash
- Lunch: Zucchini Noodles with Pesto
- Dinner: Spinach and Artichoke Stuffed Bell Peppers
- Snacks: Greek Tzatziki Dip
- Dessert: Lemon Sorbet

Day 14:

- Breakfast: Creamy Porridge with Almonds
- Lunch: Cauliflower and Chickpea Curry
- Dinner: Creamy Tomato Basil Pasta
- Snacks: Roasted Beet Chips
- Dessert: Vegan Cheesecake

Week 3

Day 15:

- Breakfast: Spinach and Feta Frittata
- Lunch: Spinach and Goat Cheese Salad
- Dinner: Vegan Shepherd's Pie
- Snacks: Avocado Salsa
- Dessert: Mixed Berry Parfait

Day 16:

- Breakfast: Baked Apple Cinnamon Oatmeal
- Lunch: Baked Falafel with Tahini Sauce
- Dinner: Cauliflower Steak with Chimichurri
- Snacks: Quinoa and Black Bean Stuffed Peppers
- Dessert: Carrot Cake Muffins

Day 17:

- Breakfast: Buckwheat Pancakes with Berries
- Lunch: Eggplant Parmesan
- Dinner: Beet and Goat Cheese Risotto
- Snacks: Sweet Potato Bites with Avocado Cream
- Dessert: Chocolate Zucchini Bread

Day 18:

- Breakfast: Veggie Breakfast Skillet
- Lunch: Minestrone Soup
- Dinner: Roasted Red Pepper and Chickpea Stew
- Snacks: Mini Vegetable Frittatas
- Dessert: Peanut Butter Banana Ice Cream

Day 19:

- Breakfast: Nutrient-Packed Smoothie Bowl
- Lunch: Chickpea and Avocado Salad
- Dinner: Mushroom and Spinach Stuffed Shells
- Snacks: Guacamole and Veggie Sticks
- Dessert: Berry and Banana Ice Cream

Day 20:

- Breakfast: Spinach and Mushroom Omelette
- Lunch: Lentil Soup with Spinach
- Dinner: Vegan Chili
- Snacks: Roasted Red Pepper Hummus
- Dessert: Chocolate Avocado Mousse

Day 21:

- Breakfast: Quinoa Breakfast Bowl
- Lunch: Caprese Quinoa Salad
- Dinner: Ratatouille
- Snacks: Edamame with Sea Salt
- Dessert: Vegan Rice Pudding

Week 4

Day 22:

- Breakfast: Blueberry Chia Pudding
- Lunch: Roasted Veggie Wrap
- Dinner: Lemon Herb Baked Tofu
- Snacks: Cucumber and Tomato Bruschetta
- Dessert: Apple Cinnamon Crisp

Day 23:

- Breakfast: Vegetable Breakfast Burrito
- Lunch: Black Bean and Corn Salad
- Dinner: Spinach and Ricotta Cannelloni
- Snacks: Baked Sweet Potato Fries
- Dessert: Chia Seed Pudding with Berries

Day 24:

- Breakfast: Oatmeal with Fresh Berries
- Lunch: Spinach and Mushroom Quesadilla
- Dinner: Sweet Potato and Lentil Curry
- Snacks: Stuffed Mushrooms
- Dessert: Baked Pears with Cinnamon

Day 25:

- Breakfast: Greek Yogurt Parfait
- Lunch: Mediterranean Farro Salad
- Dinner: Butternut Squash Risotto
- Snacks: Spinach and Artichoke Dip
- Dessert: Vegan Chocolate Chip Cookies

Day 26:

- Breakfast: Avocado Toast with Poached Egg
- Lunch: Sweet Potato and Black Bean Bowl
- Dinner: Portobello Mushroom Steaks
- Snacks: Mixed Nuts and Dried Fruit
- Dessert: Blueberry Oat Bars

Day 27:

- Breakfast: Banana Walnut Pancakes
- Lunch: Tofu Stir-Fry
- Dinner: Black Bean Enchiladas
- Snacks: Caprese Skewers
- Dessert: Coconut Mango Sorbet

Day 28:

- Breakfast: Tofu Scramble
- Lunch: Greek Salad with Tzatziki Dressing
- Dinner: Thai Vegetable Green Curry
- Snacks: Vegan Spring Rolls with Peanut Sauce
- Dessert: Chocolate Covered Strawberries

Day 29:

- Breakfast: Breakfast Quiche
- Lunch: Quinoa and Vegetable Stuffed Peppers
- Dinner: Eggplant Rollatini
- Snacks: Deviled Eggs (Vegan)
- Dessert: Pumpkin Pie Smoothie

Day 30:

- Breakfast: Coconut Mango Rice Pudding
- Lunch: Tomato Basil Soup
- Dinner: Quinoa Stuffed Acorn Squash
- Snacks: Spicy Chickpea Snack
- Dessert: Almond Joy Energy Bites

This completes the 30-day meal plan. Feel free to adapt it to your dietary needs and preferences, and enjoy your delicious and nutritious meals!

Chapter 2: Breakfast Recipes

Start your day with a burst of flavor and nutrition! In this chapter, we'll explore a delightful array of breakfast recipes designed to tantalize your taste buds while keeping your kidney health in mind. These recipes are packed with wholesome ingredients and easy-to-follow instructions to make your mornings brighter and healthier.

Nutrient-Packed Smoothie Bowl

Ingredients:

- 1 cup of fresh spinach leaves
- 1/2 cup of sliced bananas
- 1/4 cup of Greek yogurt
- 1 tablespoon of chia seeds
- 1/4 cup of almond milk
- 1 tablespoon of honey

Instructions:

1. Blend spinach, banana, yogurt, chia seeds, and almond milk until smooth.

2. Pour into a bowl, drizzle with honey, and add your favorite toppings.

Spinach and Mushroom Omelette

Ingredients:

- 2 eggs
- 1/4 cup of chopped spinach
- 1/4 cup of sliced mushrooms
- 1 tablespoon of olive oil
- Salt and pepper to taste

Instructions:

1. Heat olive oil in a pan, add spinach and mushrooms, and sauté until tender.
2. Whisk eggs, season with salt and pepper, and pour over the veggies.
3. Cook until set and fold the omelette in half.

Quinoa Breakfast Bowl

Ingredients:

- 1 cup of cooked quinoa

- 1/2 cup of mixed berries
- 2 tablespoons of chopped nuts (e.g., almonds or walnuts)
- 1 tablespoon of honey

Instructions:

1. Place cooked quinoa in a bowl.
2. Top with mixed berries, nuts, and drizzle honey over it.

Blueberry Chia Pudding

Ingredients:

- 2 tablespoons of chia seeds
- 1/2 cup of almond milk
- 1/4 cup of blueberries
- 1/2 teaspoon of vanilla extract
- 1/2 teaspoon of honey

Instructions:

1. Mix chia seeds, almond milk, vanilla extract, and honey in a jar.

2. Stir well, refrigerate overnight, and top with blueberries before serving.

Vegetable Breakfast Burrito

Ingredients:

- 1 whole-grain tortilla
- 2 scrambled eggs
- 1/4 cup of diced bell peppers
- 1/4 cup of diced tomatoes
- 2 tablespoons of shredded cheese
- Salsa for topping (optional)

Instructions:

1. Lay out the tortilla, add scrambled eggs, bell peppers, tomatoes, and cheese.
2. Roll it up, and if desired, serve with salsa.

Oatmeal with Fresh Berries

Ingredients:

- 1/2 cup of rolled oats
- 1 cup of almond milk

- 1/4 cup of fresh berries
- 1 tablespoon of honey

Instructions:

1. Cook oats with almond milk until creamy.
2. Top with fresh berries and drizzle honey over it.

Greek Yogurt Parfait

Ingredients:

- 1/2 cup of Greek yogurt
- 1/4 cup of granola
- 1/4 cup of mixed fruit (e.g., strawberries, blueberries)

Instructions:

1. Layer Greek yogurt, granola, and mixed fruit in a glass or bowl.

Avocado Toast with Poached Egg

Ingredients:

- 1 slice of whole-grain bread

- 1/2 ripe avocado

- 1 poached egg

- Salt and pepper to taste

Instructions:

1. Toast the bread, spread avocado on top, and season with salt and pepper.

2. Place the poached egg on the avocado.

Banana Walnut Pancakes

Ingredients:

- 1/2 cup of mashed bananas

- 1/4 cup of chopped walnuts

- 1/2 cup of whole-wheat flour

- 1/2 cup of almond milk

- 1 tablespoon of honey

Instructions:

1. Mix mashed bananas, chopped walnuts, whole-wheat flour, almond milk, and honey in a bowl.

2. Cook pancakes on a griddle until golden brown on both sides.

Tofu Scramble

Ingredients:

- 1/2 cup of crumbled tofu
- 1/4 cup of diced bell peppers
- 1/4 cup of diced onions
- 1/4 cup of spinach leaves
- 1/2 teaspoon of turmeric
- Salt and pepper to taste

Instructions:

1. Heat a skillet, add tofu, bell peppers, onions, and turmeric.
2. Sauté until vegetables are tender, season with salt and pepper, and stir in spinach.

Breakfast Quiche

Ingredients:

- 1 whole-grain pie crust
- 4 eggs
- 1/2 cup of chopped spinach
- 1/4 cup of diced tomatoes

- 1/4 cup of shredded cheese
- Salt and pepper to taste

Instructions:

1. Preheat the oven. Lay out the pie crust.
2. Whisk eggs, add spinach, tomatoes, cheese, salt, and pepper.
3. Pour the mixture into the pie crust and bake until set.

Coconut Mango Rice Pudding

Ingredients:

- 1/2 cup of cooked rice
- 1/4 cup of diced mango
- 2 tablespoons of shredded coconut
- 1 tablespoon of honey

Instructions:

1. Mix cooked rice, diced mango, shredded coconut, and honey in a bowl.
2. Serve warm or chilled.

Sweet Potato Hash

Ingredients:

- 1 cup of diced sweet potatoes
- 1/4 cup of diced onions
- 1/4 cup of diced bell peppers
- 1/4 cup of black beans
- 1/2 teaspoon of paprika
- Salt and pepper to taste

Instructions:

1. Heat a skillet, add sweet potatoes, onions, and bell peppers.
2. Sauté until sweet potatoes are tender, stir in black beans, paprika, salt, and pepper.

Creamy Porridge with Almonds

Ingredients:

- 1/2 cup of steel-cut oats
- 1 cup of almond milk
- 1/4 cup of chopped almonds
- 1/2 teaspoon of cinnamon

- 1 tablespoon of honey

Instructions:

1. Cook steel-cut oats with almond milk until creamy.

2. Top with chopped almonds, cinnamon, and drizzle honey over it.

Spinach and Feta Frittata

Ingredients:

- 4 eggs
- 1/2 cup of chopped spinach
- 1/4 cup of crumbled feta cheese
- Salt and pepper to taste

Instructions:

1. Whisk eggs, add chopped spinach, feta cheese, salt, and pepper.

2. Cook in an ovenproof skillet until set, then broil until golden.

Baked Apple Cinnamon Oatmeal

Ingredients:

- 1 cup of rolled oats
- 1 cup of almond milk
- 1/2 cup of diced apples
- 1/2 teaspoon of cinnamon
- 1 tablespoon of maple syrup

Instructions:

1. Mix rolled oats, almond milk, diced apples, cinnamon, and maple syrup in a baking dish.
2. Bake until oats are tender.

Buckwheat Pancakes with Berries

Ingredients:

- 1/2 cup of buckwheat flour
- 1/2 cup of almond milk
- 1/4 cup of mixed berries
- 1 tablespoon of honey

Instructions:

1. Combine buckwheat flour and almond milk, then fold in mixed berries and honey.
2. Cook pancakes on a griddle until browned.

Veggie Breakfast Skillet

Ingredients:

- 2 eggs
- 1/4 cup of diced bell peppers
- 1/4 cup of diced zucchini
- 1/4 cup of diced tomatoes
- Salt and pepper to taste

Instructions:

1. Heat a skillet, add eggs, bell peppers, zucchini, tomatoes, salt, and pepper.
2. Cook until eggs are set, stirring occasionally.

Chapter 3: Lunch Recipes

In this chapter, we're diving into a delightful array of lunch recipes that are not only delicious but also kidney-friendly. These recipes are designed to provide you with wholesome and satisfying midday meals that align with your dietary needs. Let's explore a diverse range of flavors and ingredients to keep your lunches exciting and nourishing.

Chickpea and Avocado Salad

Ingredients:

- 1 can chickpeas, drained and rinsed
- 1 ripe avocado, diced
- 1 cup cherry tomatoes, halved
- 1/4 red onion, finely chopped
- 2 tablespoons fresh cilantro, chopped
- 1 tablespoon olive oil
- Juice of 1 lemon
- Salt and pepper to taste

Instructions:

1. In a large bowl, combine chickpeas, avocado, cherry tomatoes, red onion, and cilantro.
2. Drizzle olive oil and lemon juice over the mixture.
3. Season with salt and pepper.
4. Gently toss to combine.
5. Serve chilled.

Lentil Soup with Spinach

Ingredients:

- 1 cup green or brown lentils
- 1 onion, diced
- 2 carrots, diced
- 2 celery stalks, diced
- 3 cloves garlic, minced
- 6 cups vegetable broth
- 2 cups fresh spinach, chopped
- 1 teaspoon cumin
- 1/2 teaspoon paprika
- Salt and pepper to taste

Instructions:

1. In a large pot, sauté onions, carrots, and celery until softened.
2. Add garlic, cumin, and paprika. Cook for another minute.
3. Add lentils and vegetable broth.
4. Simmer for 20-25 minutes until lentils are tender.
5. Stir in chopped spinach and cook until wilted.
6. Season with salt and pepper.
7. Serve hot.

Caprese Quinoa Salad

Ingredients:

- 1 cup quinoa, cooked and cooled
- 1 cup cherry tomatoes, halved
- 1 cup fresh mozzarella balls
- 1/4 cup fresh basil leaves, chopped
- 2 tablespoons balsamic vinegar
- 2 tablespoons olive oil
- Salt and pepper to taste

Instructions:

1. In a bowl, combine quinoa, cherry tomatoes, fresh mozzarella, and basil.
2. Drizzle with balsamic vinegar and olive oil.
3. Season with salt and pepper.
4. Gently toss to combine.
5. Serve at room temperature.

Roasted Veggie Wrap

Ingredients:

- 1 cup mixed roasted vegetables (bell peppers, zucchini, eggplant, etc.)
- 2 whole-grain tortillas
- 1/4 cup hummus
- 1/4 cup fresh spinach leaves
- 2 tablespoons feta cheese (optional)
- Salt and pepper to taste

Instructions:

1. Lay out tortillas and spread hummus evenly over each.
2. Place roasted vegetables on top.

3. Add fresh spinach leaves and feta cheese if desired.

4. Season with salt and pepper.

5. Roll up tightly and slice in half.

6. Serve as wraps.

Black Bean and Corn Salad

Ingredients:

- 1 can black beans, drained and rinsed
- 1 cup corn kernels (fresh or frozen, thawed)
- 1 red bell pepper, diced
- 1/4 cup red onion, finely chopped
- 2 tablespoons fresh cilantro, chopped
- 2 tablespoons lime juice
- 1 tablespoon olive oil
- Salt and pepper to taste

Instructions:

1. In a large bowl, combine black beans, corn, red bell pepper, red onion, and cilantro.

2. Drizzle with lime juice and olive oil.

3. Season with salt and pepper.

4. Gently toss to combine.

5. Serve chilled.

Spinach and Mushroom Quesadilla

Ingredients:

- 2 whole-grain tortillas
- 1 cup fresh spinach leaves
- 1 cup mushrooms, sliced
- 1/2 cup shredded mozzarella cheese
- 1/4 cup red onion, finely chopped
- 1 clove garlic, minced
- 1/2 teaspoon olive oil
- Salt and pepper to taste

Instructions:

1. In a skillet, heat olive oil over medium heat.
2. Add mushrooms, red onion, and garlic. Sauté until mushrooms are tender.
3. Lay out tortillas and sprinkle half of the shredded mozzarella on each.
4. Place a layer of fresh spinach leaves on top.
5. Spoon the sautéed mushroom mixture onto one side of each tortilla.

6. Fold the tortillas in half.

7. Heat a non-stick skillet and cook quesadillas until cheese is melted and tortillas are golden brown.

8. Slice and serve hot.

Mediterranean Farro Salad

Ingredients:

- 1 cup farro, cooked and cooled
- 1/2 cucumber, diced
- 1 cup cherry tomatoes, halved
- 1/4 cup Kalamata olives, pitted and sliced
- 1/4 cup red onion, finely chopped
- 1/4 cup feta cheese, crumbled (optional)
- 2 tablespoons fresh parsley, chopped
- 2 tablespoons olive oil
- 2 tablespoons red wine vinegar
- Salt and pepper to taste

Instructions:

1. In a large bowl, combine cooked farro, cucumber, cherry tomatoes, Kalamata olives, red onion, and feta cheese (if using).

2. In a separate small bowl, whisk together olive oil and
    red wine vinegar.

3. Drizzle the dressing over the salad.

4. Add fresh parsley and season with salt and pepper.

5. Gently toss to combine.

6. Serve chilled.

Sweet Potato and Black Bean Bowl

Ingredients:

- 2 sweet potatoes, peeled and cubed
- 1 can black beans, drained and rinsed
- 1 cup cooked quinoa
- 1/2 avocado, sliced
- 1/4 cup fresh cilantro, chopped
- Juice of 1 lime
- 1 tablespoon olive oil
- Salt and pepper to taste

Instructions:

1. Preheat the oven to 400°F (200°C).

2. Toss sweet potato cubes with olive oil, salt, and
    pepper.

3. Roast sweet potatoes for 20-25 minutes until tender and slightly crispy.

4. In a bowl, combine black beans, cooked quinoa, roasted sweet potatoes, and avocado slices.

5. Drizzle with lime juice.

6. Garnish with fresh cilantro.

7. Serve warm.

Tofu Stir-Fry

Ingredients:

- 1 block extra-firm tofu, cubed
- 2 cups mixed vegetables (broccoli, bell peppers, snap peas, etc.), chopped
- 2 tablespoons soy sauce
- 1 tablespoon sesame oil
- 1 tablespoon ginger, minced
- 2 cloves garlic, minced
- 1 tablespoon cornstarch
- 2 tablespoons water
- Rice or quinoa for serving

Instructions:

1. Press tofu to remove excess water and cut into cubes.

2. In a small bowl, whisk together soy sauce, sesame oil, ginger, garlic, cornstarch, and water to make the sauce.

3. Heat a large skillet or wok over medium-high heat and add tofu cubes.

4. Stir-fry tofu until lightly browned on all sides, then remove from the pan and set aside.

5. In the same pan, add mixed vegetables and stir-fry until they begin to soften.

6. Return tofu to the pan, pour the sauce over everything, and stir-fry until well coated and heated through.

7. Serve over rice or quinoa.

Greek Salad with Tzatziki Dressing

Ingredients:

- 2 cups cucumber, diced
- 2 cups cherry tomatoes, halved
- 1 cup Kalamata olives, pitted
- 1/2 cup red onion, thinly sliced

- 1/2 cup feta cheese, crumbled
- 2 tablespoons fresh dill, chopped
- 1/4 cup Greek yogurt
- 1/4 cup sour cream
- 2 tablespoons lemon juice
- 1 clove garlic, minced
- Salt and pepper to taste

Instructions:

1. In a large bowl, combine cucumber, cherry tomatoes, Kalamata olives, red onion, feta cheese, and fresh dill.
2. In a separate bowl, whisk together Greek yogurt, sour cream, lemon juice, garlic, salt, and pepper to make the dressing.
3. Drizzle the dressing over the salad and toss to coat.
4. Serve chilled.

Quinoa and Vegetable Stuffed Peppers

Ingredients:

- 4 bell peppers, any color
- 1 cup quinoa, cooked
- 1 cup mixed vegetables (zucchini, carrots, corn, etc.), diced
- 1 can black beans, drained and rinsed
- 1/2 cup tomato sauce
- 1 teaspoon cumin
- 1/2 teaspoon chili powder
- Salt and pepper to taste
- Shredded cheddar cheese (optional)

Instructions:

1. Preheat the oven to 375°F (190°C).
2. Cut the tops off the bell peppers and remove the seeds and membranes.
3. In a bowl, combine cooked quinoa, mixed vegetables, black beans, tomato sauce, cumin, chili powder, salt, and pepper.
4. Stuff the mixture into the bell peppers.

5. Place the stuffed peppers in a baking dish and cover with aluminum foil.

6. Bake for 30-35 minutes until peppers are tender.

7. If desired, sprinkle with shredded cheddar cheese and bake for an additional 5 minutes until cheese is melted.

8. Serve hot.

Tomato Basil Soup

Ingredients:

- 6 ripe tomatoes, chopped
- 1 onion, chopped
- 3 cloves garlic, minced
- 4 cups vegetable broth
- 1/4 cup fresh basil leaves, chopped
- 2 tablespoons olive oil
- Salt and pepper to taste
- Croutons for garnish (optional)

Instructions:

1. In a large pot, heat olive oil over medium heat.

2. Add chopped onion and garlic, sauté until fragrant.

3. Add chopped tomatoes and cook until they begin to break down.

4. Pour in vegetable broth and bring to a simmer.

5. Let the soup simmer for about 20 minutes.

6. Stir in fresh basil.

7. Using an immersion blender, blend the soup until smooth.

8. Season with salt and pepper.

9. Serve hot, garnished with croutons if desired.

Zucchini Noodles with Pesto

Ingredients:

- 2 large zucchinis, spiralized into noodles
- 1/2 cup cherry tomatoes, halved
- 1/4 cup pine nuts, toasted
- 1/4 cup fresh basil pesto (store-bought or homemade)
- Grated Parmesan cheese (optional)
- Salt and pepper to taste

Instructions:

1. Spiralize zucchinis into noodles and set aside.

2. In a large skillet, heat a small amount of olive oil over medium heat.

3. Add zucchini noodles and cherry tomatoes, sauté for 2-3 minutes until just tender.

4. Stir in fresh basil pesto and toasted pine nuts.

5. Season with salt and pepper.

6. Serve hot, garnished with grated Parmesan cheese if desired.

Cauliflower and Chickpea Curry

Ingredients:

- 1 small cauliflower, cut into florets
- 1 can chickpeas, drained and rinsed
- 1 onion, chopped
- 3 cloves garlic, minced
- 1 can diced tomatoes
- 1 can coconut milk
- 2 tablespoons curry powder
- 1 teaspoon cumin
- 1 teaspoon turmeric
- Salt and pepper to taste
- Fresh cilantro for garnish

Instructions:

1. In a large pot, sauté onions and garlic until translucent.
2. Add curry powder, cumin, turmeric, salt, and pepper. Cook for 2 minutes.
3. Add cauliflower florets, chickpeas, diced tomatoes, and coconut milk.
4. Simmer for 20-25 minutes until cauliflower is tender.
5. Serve hot, garnished with fresh cilantro.

Spinach and Goat Cheese Salad

Ingredients:

- 4 cups fresh spinach leaves
- 1/2 cup goat cheese, crumbled
- 1/4 cup walnuts, chopped and toasted
- 1/4 cup dried cranberries
- Balsamic vinaigrette dressing
- Salt and pepper to taste

Instructions:

1. In a large bowl, combine fresh spinach, crumbled goat cheese, toasted walnuts, and dried cranberries.

2. Drizzle with balsamic vinaigrette dressing.

3. Season with salt and pepper.

4. Gently toss to combine.

5. Serve chilled.

Baked Falafel with Tahini Sauce

Ingredients:

For the Falafel:

- 1 can chickpeas, drained and rinsed
- 1/4 cup fresh parsley, chopped
- 1/4 cup onion, chopped
- 2 cloves garlic, minced
- 1 teaspoon ground cumin
- 1 teaspoon ground coriander
- 1/4 teaspoon cayenne pepper
- Salt and pepper to taste
- 2 tablespoons olive oil (for brushing)

For the Tahini Sauce:

- 1/4 cup tahini
- 2 tablespoons lemon juice
- 2 tablespoons water

- 1 clove garlic, minced
- Salt to taste

Instructions:

For the Falafel:

1. Preheat the oven to 375°F (190°C).
2. In a food processor, combine chickpeas, parsley, onion, garlic, cumin, coriander, cayenne pepper, salt, and pepper.
3. Pulse until the mixture is finely chopped but not pureed.
4. Shape the mixture into small patties and place them on a baking sheet.
5. Brush the tops with olive oil.
6. Bake for 15-20 minutes, flipping the falafel halfway through until they are golden brown and firm.

For the Tahini Sauce:

1. In a small bowl, whisk together tahini, lemon juice, water, minced garlic, and salt.
2. Adjust the consistency with more water if needed.

Eggplant Parmesan

Ingredients:

- 1 large eggplant, sliced into rounds
- 1 cup breadcrumbs (use panko for extra crispiness)
- 1 cup marinara sauce
- 1 cup mozzarella cheese, shredded
- 1/4 cup Parmesan cheese, grated
- 1/4 cup fresh basil leaves, chopped
- Olive oil for frying
- Salt and pepper to taste

Instructions:

1. Preheat the oven to 375°F (190°C).
2. Heat olive oil in a skillet over medium heat.
3. Dip eggplant slices in breadcrumbs, coating both sides.
4. Fry eggplant slices until golden brown and crispy, then drain on paper towels.
5. In a baking dish, spread a thin layer of marinara sauce.
6. Place a layer of fried eggplant slices over the sauce.

7. Sprinkle mozzarella and Parmesan cheese over the eggplant.

8. Repeat the layers until all ingredients are used, ending with cheese on top.

9. Bake for 25-30 minutes until cheese is bubbly and golden.

10. Garnish with fresh basil leaves before serving.

Minestrone Soup

Ingredients:

- 1 cup small pasta (e.g., elbow or small shells)
- 1 can kidney beans, drained and rinsed
- 1 can diced tomatoes
- 2 carrots, diced
- 2 celery stalks, diced
- 1 onion, chopped
- 2 cloves garlic, minced
- 6 cups vegetable broth
- 1 teaspoon Italian seasoning
- Salt and pepper to taste
- Grated Parmesan cheese (optional)

Instructions:

1. In a large pot, sauté onions, carrots, and celery until softened.
2. Add garlic and cook for another minute.
3. Pour in vegetable broth and diced tomatoes.
4. Bring to a simmer and add pasta.
5. Cook until pasta is tender.
6. Stir in kidney beans and Italian seasoning.
7. Season with salt and pepper.
8. Serve hot, garnished with grated Parmesan cheese if desired.

Chapter 4: Dinner Recipes

In this chapter, we present an array of delectable dinner recipes that cater to both your taste buds and your kidney health. These dishes are thoughtfully crafted to be nutritious, kidney-friendly, and bursting with flavor. So, let's dive into the culinary world of kidney-conscious dinners:

Mushroom and Spinach Stuffed Shells

Ingredients:

- 12 jumbo pasta shells
- 2 cups fresh spinach, chopped
- 1 ½ cups mushrooms, finely chopped
- 1 cup ricotta cheese
- ½ cup shredded mozzarella cheese
- 1 egg
- 1 cup marinara sauce
- Salt and pepper to taste

Instructions:

1. Cook pasta shells according to package instructions. Drain and set aside.
2. In a skillet, sauté mushrooms and spinach until tender. Remove from heat and let cool.
3. In a mixing bowl, combine ricotta, mozzarella, egg, sautéed mushrooms, and spinach. Season with salt and pepper.
4. Preheat your oven to 375°F (190°C).
5. Stuff each cooked pasta shell with the mushroom and spinach mixture.
6. Spread a thin layer of marinara sauce in a baking dish. Place the stuffed shells in the dish.
7. Pour the remaining marinara sauce over the shells.
8. Cover with foil and bake for 25 minutes. Remove foil and bake for an additional 10 minutes until bubbly and golden.

Vegan Chili

Ingredients:

- 1 cup dried black beans, soaked and cooked
- 1 cup kidney beans, canned and drained

- 1 cup corn kernels
- 1 bell pepper, diced
- 1 onion, chopped
- 3 cloves garlic, minced
- 1 can diced tomatoes
- 2 cups vegetable broth
- 2 tablespoons chili powder
- 1 teaspoon cumin
- Salt and pepper to taste
- Optional toppings: avocado, cilantro, lime wedges

Instructions:

1. In a large pot, sauté onions and garlic until fragrant.
2. Add bell pepper and cook until slightly softened.
3. Stir in chili powder and cumin.
4. Add cooked black beans, kidney beans, corn, diced tomatoes, and vegetable broth.
5. Bring to a boil, then reduce heat and simmer for 20-25 minutes.
6. Season with salt and pepper to taste.
7. Serve with your choice of toppings.

Ratatouille

Ingredients:

- 1 eggplant, diced
- 2 zucchinis, diced
- 1 bell pepper, diced
- 1 onion, chopped
- 2 cloves garlic, minced
- 2 cups diced tomatoes
- 2 tablespoons olive oil
- 1 teaspoon dried thyme
- Salt and pepper to taste
- Fresh basil for garnish

Instructions:

1. In a large skillet, heat olive oil over medium heat.
2. Add onions and garlic, sauté until fragrant.
3. Layer the diced eggplant, zucchini, and bell pepper on top.
4. Pour diced tomatoes over the vegetables. Sprinkle with thyme, salt, and pepper.
5. Cover and simmer for 25-30 minutes, stirring occasionally.

6. Garnish with fresh basil before serving.

Lemon Herb Baked Tofu

Ingredients:

- 1 block of extra-firm tofu, pressed and cubed
- 2 tablespoons olive oil
- 2 tablespoons lemon juice
- 1 teaspoon dried basil
- 1 teaspoon dried thyme
- Salt and pepper to taste
- Lemon zest for garnish

Instructions:

1. Preheat your oven to 375°F (190°C). Grease a baking dish.
2. In a small bowl, whisk together olive oil, lemon juice, basil, thyme, salt, and pepper.
3. Place the cubed tofu in the baking dish.
4. Pour the lemon herb mixture over the tofu, making sure it's well coated.
5. Bake for 20-25 minutes or until tofu is golden and slightly crispy.

6. Garnish with lemon zest before serving.

Spinach and Ricotta Cannelloni

Ingredients:

- 8 cannelloni tubes
- 2 cups fresh spinach, chopped
- 1 cup ricotta cheese
- ½ cup grated Parmesan cheese
- 1 egg
- 1 cup marinara sauce
- Salt and pepper to taste

Instructions:

1. Cook cannelloni tubes according to package instructions. Drain and set aside.
2. In a mixing bowl, combine chopped spinach, ricotta, Parmesan, egg, salt, and pepper.
3. Preheat your oven to 375°F (190°C).
4. Stuff each cannelloni tube with the spinach and ricotta mixture.
5. Spread a thin layer of marinara sauce in a baking dish. Place the stuffed cannelloni in the dish.

6. Pour the remaining marinara sauce over the cannelloni.

7. Cover with foil and bake for 20-25 minutes. Remove foil and bake for an additional 10 minutes until bubbly.

Sweet Potato and Lentil Curry

Ingredients:

- 2 sweet potatoes, peeled and diced
- 1 cup red lentils
- 1 onion, chopped
- 2 cloves garlic, minced
- 1 can coconut milk
- 2 tablespoons curry powder
- 1 teaspoon turmeric
- Salt and pepper to taste
- Fresh cilantro for garnish

Instructions:

1. In a large pot, sauté onions and garlic until fragrant.

2. Add curry powder and turmeric, and stir for a minute.

3. Add sweet potatoes, red lentils, and coconut milk.

4. Bring to a boil, then reduce heat and simmer for 20-25 minutes until sweet potatoes and lentils are tender.

5. Season with salt and pepper.

6. Garnish with fresh cilantro before serving.

Butternut Squash Risotto

Ingredients:

- 2 cups Arborio rice
- 1 small butternut squash, peeled and diced
- 1 onion, chopped
- 3 cups vegetable broth
- 1 cup dry white wine
- 2 tablespoons olive oil
- 1 teaspoon dried sage
- Salt and pepper to taste
- Grated Parmesan cheese (optional)

Instructions:

1. In a large skillet, heat olive oil over medium heat.

2. Add onions and cook until translucent.

3. Add Arborio rice and stir for a couple of minutes.

4. Pour in the white wine and let it simmer until mostly absorbed.

5. Begin adding vegetable broth, one ladle at a time, stirring until absorbed before adding more.

6. After about 15 minutes, add the butternut squash and continue to cook until rice is creamy and squash is tender.

7. Stir in dried sage, salt, and pepper.

8. Serve with grated Parmesan cheese if desired.

Portobello Mushroom Steaks

Ingredients:

- 4 large Portobello mushrooms
- 2 tablespoons balsamic vinegar
- 2 tablespoons olive oil
- 2 cloves garlic, minced
- 1 teaspoon dried rosemary
- Salt and pepper to taste

Instructions:

1. Preheat your grill or grill pan to medium-high heat.

2. In a small bowl, whisk together balsamic vinegar, olive oil, garlic, rosemary, salt, and pepper.

3. Brush the Portobello mushrooms with the mixture.

4. Grill mushrooms for about 5-7 minutes on each side until tender and grill marks appear.

5. Serve as a steak alternative with your favorite sides.

Black Bean Enchiladas

Ingredients:

- 8 whole wheat tortillas
- 2 cans black beans, drained and rinsed
- 1 onion, chopped
- 2 cloves garlic, minced
- 1 red bell pepper, diced
- 1 teaspoon cumin
- 1 teaspoon chili powder
- 1 cup enchilada sauce
- 1 cup shredded cheese (optional)
- Chopped fresh cilantro for garnish

Instructions:

1. Preheat your oven to 350°F (175°C).

2. In a skillet, sauté onions, garlic, and red bell pepper until softened.

3. Add black beans, cumin, and chili powder. Cook for a few minutes.

4. Place a portion of the bean mixture in each tortilla, roll them up, and place them seam-side down in a baking dish.

5. Pour enchilada sauce over the tortillas. Sprinkle with cheese if desired.

6. Bake for 20-25 minutes until bubbly and cheese is melted.

7. Garnish with chopped cilantro before serving.

Thai Vegetable Green Curry

Ingredients:

- 1 can coconut milk
- 2 tablespoons green curry paste
- 2 cups mixed vegetables (e.g., broccoli, bell peppers, carrots)
- 1 block of firm tofu, cubed
- 2 tablespoons soy sauce
- 1 tablespoon brown sugar

- Fresh basil leaves for garnish
- Cooked rice for serving

Instructions:

1. In a large pan, heat coconut milk and green curry paste over medium heat.
2. Add mixed vegetables and tofu.
3. Stir in soy sauce and brown sugar.
4. Simmer for 15-20 minutes until vegetables are tender.
5. Serve over cooked rice and garnish with fresh basil leaves.

Eggplant Rollatini

Ingredients:

- 2 large eggplants, thinly sliced lengthwise
- 2 cups ricotta cheese
- 1 cup shredded mozzarella cheese
- 1 egg
- 1 cup marinara sauce
- Salt and pepper to taste
- Fresh basil for garnish

Instructions:

1. Preheat your oven to 375°F (190°C).

2. In a bowl, combine ricotta, mozzarella, egg, salt, and pepper.

3. Spread a thin layer of marinara sauce in a baking dish.

4. Place a spoonful of the ricotta mixture on each eggplant slice, roll them up, and place them in the dish.

5. Pour the remaining marinara sauce over the rollatini.

6. Bake for 25-30 minutes until bubbly and golden.

7. Garnish with fresh basil before serving.

Quinoa Stuffed Acorn Squash

Ingredients:

- 2 acorn squashes, halved and seeds removed
- 1 cup quinoa, cooked
- 1 cup black beans, canned and drained
- 1 cup diced tomatoes
- 1/2 cup corn kernels
- 1/2 cup diced bell pepper (red or yellow)
- 1 teaspoon cumin

- 1/2 teaspoon chili powder
- Salt and pepper to taste
- Fresh cilantro for garnish

Instructions:

1. Preheat your oven to 375°F (190°C).
2. Place acorn squash halves on a baking sheet, cut side up.
3. Roast for about 30-40 minutes or until the squash is tender.
4. In a large bowl, combine cooked quinoa, black beans, diced tomatoes, corn, bell pepper, cumin, chili powder, salt, and pepper.
5. Stuff each acorn squash half with the quinoa mixture.
6. Return to the oven for another 15 minutes.
7. Garnish with fresh cilantro before serving.

Spinach and Artichoke Stuffed Bell Peppers

Ingredients:

- 4 bell peppers, tops removed and seeds removed

- 2 cups fresh spinach, chopped
- 1 cup artichoke hearts, chopped
- 1 cup cooked brown rice
- 1/2 cup shredded mozzarella cheese
- 1/2 cup grated Parmesan cheese
- Salt and pepper to taste
- Marinara sauce for serving

Instructions:

1. Preheat your oven to 375°F (190°C).
2. In a bowl, combine chopped spinach, artichoke hearts, cooked brown rice, mozzarella cheese, Parmesan cheese, salt, and pepper.
3. Stuff each bell pepper with the spinach and artichoke mixture.
4. Place the stuffed peppers in a baking dish.
5. Bake for 25-30 minutes or until peppers are tender and filling is heated through.
6. Serve with marinara sauce.

Creamy Tomato Basil Pasta

Ingredients:

- 8 oz whole wheat pasta
- 1 can diced tomatoes
- 1/2 cup heavy cream (or a dairy-free alternative)
- 1/4 cup fresh basil leaves, chopped
- 2 cloves garlic, minced
- Salt and pepper to taste
- Grated Parmesan cheese (optional)

Instructions:

1. Cook pasta according to package instructions. Drain and set aside.
2. In a saucepan, combine diced tomatoes, heavy cream, garlic, salt, and pepper.
3. Simmer for 5-7 minutes until slightly thickened.
4. Stir in fresh basil.
5. Toss the cooked pasta in the creamy tomato basil sauce.
6. Serve with grated Parmesan cheese if desired.

Vegan Shepherd's Pie

Ingredients:

- 4 cups mashed potatoes
- 1 cup lentils, cooked
- 1 cup mixed vegetables (carrots, peas, corn)
- 1 onion, chopped
- 2 cloves garlic, minced
- 1 cup vegetable broth
- 2 tablespoons tomato paste
- 1 teaspoon thyme
- Salt and pepper to taste
- Fresh parsley for garnish

Instructions:

1. Preheat your oven to 375°F (190°C).
2. In a skillet, sauté onions and garlic until softened.
3. Add cooked lentils, mixed vegetables, vegetable broth, tomato paste, thyme, salt, and pepper.
4. Simmer for 10-15 minutes until the mixture thickens.
5. Transfer the lentil and vegetable mixture to a baking dish.
6. Spread mashed potatoes on top.

7. Bake for 20-25 minutes or until the top is golden.

8. Garnish with fresh parsley before serving.

Cauliflower Steak with Chimichurri

Ingredients:

- 2 large cauliflower steaks
- 2 tablespoons olive oil
- Salt and pepper to taste

For the Chimichurri Sauce:

- 1 cup fresh parsley, chopped
- 1/4 cup fresh cilantro, chopped
- 2 cloves garlic, minced
- 1/4 cup red wine vinegar
- 1/4 cup olive oil
- Salt and pepper to taste
- Red pepper flakes (optional, for heat)

Instructions:

1. Preheat your grill or grill pan to medium-high heat.

2. Brush cauliflower steaks with olive oil and season with salt and pepper.

3. Grill cauliflower steaks for about 5-7 minutes on each side until tender and grill marks appear.

4. While grilling, prepare the chimichurri sauce by mixing all the sauce ingredients in a bowl.

5. Serve the grilled cauliflower steaks with chimichurri sauce drizzled on top.

Beet and Goat Cheese Risotto

Ingredients:

- 2 cups Arborio rice
- 4 cups vegetable broth
- 2 cups cooked beets, diced
- 1/2 cup goat cheese
- 1 onion, chopped
- 2 cloves garlic, minced
- 2 tablespoons olive oil
- Salt and pepper to taste

Instructions:

1. In a saucepan, heat vegetable broth and keep it simmering.

2. In a large skillet, heat olive oil over medium heat.

3. Add onions and garlic, sauté until translucent.

4. Stir in Arborio rice and cook for a couple of minutes.

5. Begin adding the simmering vegetable broth, one ladle at a time, stirring until absorbed before adding more.

6. After about 15-20 minutes, when the rice is creamy and cooked, fold in diced beets and goat cheese.

7. Season with salt and pepper.

8. Serve hot.

Roasted Red Pepper and Chickpea Stew

Ingredients:

- 2 red bell peppers, roasted, peeled, and chopped
- 2 cans chickpeas, drained and rinsed
- 1 onion, chopped
- 2 cloves garlic, minced
- 1 can diced tomatoes
- 2 cups vegetable broth
- 1 teaspoon smoked paprika
- Salt and pepper to taste

- Fresh parsley for garnish

Instructions:

1. In a large pot, sauté onions and garlic until fragrant.
2. Add roasted red peppers, chickpeas, diced tomatoes, vegetable broth, smoked paprika, salt, and pepper.
3. Simmer for 20-25 minutes, allowing flavors to meld.
4. Garnish with fresh parsley before serving.

Chapter 5: Snacks and Appetizers

In this chapter, we've curated a delightful selection of vegetarian snacks and appetizers that are not only delicious but also perfect for satisfying your cravings. Whether you're hosting a gathering or simply looking for a tasty bite between meals, these recipes have got you covered. Let's dive into these mouthwatering creations.

Guacamole and Veggie Sticks

Ingredients:

- 3 ripe avocados
- 1 small red onion, finely diced
- 2 cloves garlic, minced
- 1-2 tomatoes, diced
- Juice of 1 lime
- Salt and pepper to taste
- Assorted veggie sticks (carrots, celery, bell peppers)

Instructions:

1. Cut the avocados in half, remove the pit, and scoop the flesh into a bowl.
2. Mash the avocados with a fork, leaving some chunks for texture.
3. Add the diced onion, minced garlic, diced tomatoes, and lime juice. Mix well.
4. Season with salt and pepper to taste.
5. Serve the guacamole with an assortment of veggie sticks.

Roasted Red Pepper Hummus

Ingredients:

- 1 can (15 oz) chickpeas, drained and rinsed
- 2 roasted red peppers (from a jar), drained
- 3 tablespoons tahini
- 2 cloves garlic, minced
- Juice of 1 lemon
- 2 tablespoons olive oil
- Salt and paprika to taste

Instructions:

1. In a food processor, combine chickpeas, roasted red peppers, tahini, minced garlic, and lemon juice.
2. Process until smooth, scraping down the sides as needed.
3. With the processor running, drizzle in the olive oil until the hummus is creamy.
4. Season with salt and paprika to taste.
5. Serve with pita bread, crackers, or vegetable sticks.

Edamame with Sea Salt

Ingredients:

- 2 cups edamame (frozen or fresh)
- Sea salt, to taste

Instructions:

1. Steam or boil the edamame according to package instructions.
2. Drain and sprinkle with sea salt while still warm.
3. Toss to coat evenly.
4. Serve as a simple and nutritious snack.

Cucumber and Tomato Bruschetta

Ingredients:

- 4 Roma tomatoes, diced
- 1 cucumber, diced
- 1/4 red onion, finely chopped
- 2 cloves garlic, minced
- 2 tablespoons fresh basil, chopped
- 2 tablespoons balsamic vinegar
- 2 tablespoons olive oil
- Salt and pepper to taste
- Baguette slices, toasted (optional)

Instructions:

1. In a bowl, combine the diced tomatoes, cucumber, red onion, minced garlic, and fresh basil.
2. Drizzle with balsamic vinegar and olive oil. Mix gently.
3. Season with salt and pepper to taste.
4. Let the mixture sit for about 15 minutes to allow the flavors to meld.
5. Serve as a topping for toasted baguette slices or as a dip.

Baked Sweet Potato Fries

Ingredients:

- 2 large sweet potatoes, cut into fries
- 2 tablespoons olive oil
- 1 teaspoon paprika
- 1/2 teaspoon garlic powder
- 1/2 teaspoon salt
- 1/4 teaspoon black pepper

Instructions:

1. Preheat your oven to 425°F (220°C) and line a baking sheet with parchment paper.
2. In a large bowl, toss the sweet potato fries with olive oil, paprika, garlic powder, salt, and black pepper until evenly coated.
3. Arrange the fries in a single layer on the prepared baking sheet.
4. Bake for 25-30 minutes, turning once halfway through, or until the fries are crispy and golden brown.
5. Serve hot as a healthy and satisfying snack.

Stuffed Mushrooms

Ingredients:

- 12 large mushroom caps, cleaned and stems removed
- 1/2 cup cream cheese
- 1/4 cup grated Parmesan cheese
- 2 cloves garlic, minced
- 2 tablespoons fresh parsley, chopped
- Salt and black pepper to taste

Instructions:

1. Preheat your oven to 350°F (175°C) and line a baking sheet with parchment paper.
2. In a bowl, mix together cream cheese, Parmesan cheese, minced garlic, and chopped parsley. Season with salt and pepper.
3. Stuff each mushroom cap with the cream cheese mixture.
4. Arrange the stuffed mushrooms on the prepared baking sheet.
5. Bake for 20-25 minutes or until the mushrooms are tender and the filling is golden.
6. Serve these delightful bites as an appetizer.

Spinach and Artichoke Dip

Ingredients:

- 1 cup frozen chopped spinach, thawed and drained
- 1 can (14 oz) artichoke hearts, drained and chopped
- 1 cup cream cheese
- 1/2 cup sour cream
- 1/4 cup mayonnaise
- 1 cup grated mozzarella cheese
- 1/4 cup grated Parmesan cheese
- 1 clove garlic, minced
- Salt and pepper to taste

Instructions:

1. Preheat your oven to 350°F (175°C).
2. In a large bowl, combine the thawed and drained spinach, chopped artichoke hearts, cream cheese, sour cream, mayonnaise, mozzarella cheese, Parmesan cheese, minced garlic, salt, and pepper.
3. Mix well until all ingredients are fully incorporated.
4. Transfer the mixture to a baking dish and bake for about 25-30 minutes, or until it's hot and bubbly.
5. Serve with tortilla chips or bread slices for dipping.

Mixed Nuts and Dried Fruit

Ingredients:

- 1 cup mixed nuts (almonds, cashews, walnuts, etc.)
- 1/2 cup dried cranberries
- 1/2 cup dried apricots, chopped
- 1/2 cup dried figs, chopped

Instructions:

1. In a bowl, combine the mixed nuts, dried cranberries, chopped dried apricots, and chopped dried figs.
2. Toss together to create a delightful blend of sweet and nutty flavors.
3. Serve this nutritious mix as a satisfying snack.

Caprese Skewers

Ingredients:

- Cherry tomatoes
- Fresh mozzarella balls
- Fresh basil leaves
- Balsamic glaze (store-bought or homemade)
- Skewers

Instructions:

1. Thread a cherry tomato, a mozzarella ball, and a fresh basil leaf onto each skewer.
2. Arrange the skewers on a serving platter.
3. Drizzle with balsamic glaze.
4. These Caprese skewers offer a burst of fresh flavors in every bite.

Vegan Spring Rolls with Peanut Sauce

Ingredients for Spring Rolls:

- Rice paper wrappers
- Lettuce leaves
- Carrot strips
- Cucumber strips
- Fresh mint leaves
- Cooked rice vermicelli noodles
- Avocado slices
- Red bell pepper strips

Ingredients for Peanut Sauce:

- 1/4 cup peanut butter
- 2 tablespoons soy sauce
- 2 tablespoons maple syrup
- 1 tablespoon rice vinegar
- 1 clove garlic, minced
- Water (for thinning)

Instructions:

1. Dip a rice paper wrapper into warm water for a few seconds until it softens.
2. Lay the softened wrapper flat and add a lettuce leaf, carrot strips, cucumber strips, mint leaves, vermicelli noodles, avocado slices, and red bell pepper strips in the center.
3. Fold the sides of the wrapper in and roll it up tightly.
4. Repeat with the remaining ingredients to make more spring rolls.
5. For the peanut sauce, whisk together peanut butter, soy sauce, maple syrup, rice vinegar, and minced garlic. Add water as needed to achieve your desired consistency.

6. Serve the spring rolls with the peanut sauce for dipping.

Deviled Eggs (Vegan)

Ingredients:

- 6 hard-boiled eggs (use vegan alternatives if preferred)
- 2 tablespoons vegan mayonnaise
- 1 teaspoon Dijon mustard
- 1 teaspoon apple cider vinegar
- Paprika and chives for garnish

Instructions:

1. Cut the hard-boiled eggs in half and remove the yolks.
2. In a bowl, mash the yolks and mix with vegan mayonnaise, Dijon mustard, and apple cider vinegar until smooth.
3. Fill the egg whites with the yolk mixture.
4. Garnish with paprika and chopped chives.
5. These vegan deviled eggs are a cruelty-free twist on a classic appetizer.

Spicy Chickpea Snack

Ingredients:

- 1 can (15 oz) chickpeas, drained and rinsed
- 2 tablespoons olive oil
- 1 teaspoon smoked paprika
- 1/2 teaspoon cayenne pepper (adjust to taste)
- Salt to taste

Instructions:

1. Preheat your oven to 400°F (200°C) and line a baking sheet with parchment paper.
2. In a bowl, toss the chickpeas with olive oil, smoked paprika, cayenne pepper, and salt until well coated.
3. Spread the chickpeas in a single layer on the baking sheet.
4. Bake for 20-25 minutes or until they are crispy and slightly golden.
5. Allow them to cool before serving. These spicy chickpeas make for a crunchy and satisfying snack.

Greek Tzatziki Dip

Ingredients:

- 1 cup Greek yogurt
- 1/2 cucumber, grated and drained
- 2 cloves garlic, minced
- 1 tablespoon fresh dill, chopped
- 1 tablespoon fresh mint, chopped
- 1 tablespoon olive oil
- 1 teaspoon lemon juice
- Salt and pepper to taste

Instructions:

1. In a bowl, combine Greek yogurt, grated cucumber (make sure to drain excess liquid), minced garlic, chopped dill, chopped mint, olive oil, and lemon juice.
2. Mix well and season with salt and pepper to taste.
3. Refrigerate for about 30 minutes before serving.
4. Serve this refreshing dip with pita bread or vegetable sticks.

Roasted Beet Chips

Ingredients:

- 2-3 medium-sized beets, peeled and thinly sliced
- 1-2 tablespoons olive oil
- Salt and pepper to taste

Instructions:

1. Preheat your oven to 350°F (175°C).
2. In a bowl, toss the beet slices with olive oil, salt, and pepper until they are evenly coated.
3. Arrange the beet slices in a single layer on a baking sheet.
4. Bake for 20-25 minutes, or until the beet chips are crispy and slightly browned.
5. Let them cool before serving as a colorful and nutritious snack.

Avocado Salsa

Ingredients:

- 2 ripe avocados, diced
- 1 tomato, diced

- 1/4 red onion, finely chopped
- 1/4 cup fresh cilantro, chopped
- Juice of 1 lime
- Salt and pepper to taste

Instructions:

1. In a bowl, combine diced avocados, diced tomato, finely chopped red onion, chopped cilantro, lime juice, salt, and pepper.
2. Gently mix to combine all the ingredients.
3. Serve this avocado salsa as a refreshing and creamy dip or topping.

Quinoa and Black Bean Stuffed Peppers

Ingredients:

- 4 large bell peppers, any color
- 1 cup cooked quinoa
- 1 can (15 oz) black beans, drained and rinsed
- 1 cup corn kernels
- 1 cup diced tomatoes

- 1/2 teaspoon cumin
- 1/2 teaspoon chili powder
- Salt and pepper to taste
- Grated cheese (optional for topping)

Instructions:

1. Preheat your oven to 375°F (190°C).
2. Cut the tops off the bell peppers and remove the seeds.
3. In a bowl, combine cooked quinoa, black beans, corn, diced tomatoes, cumin, chili powder, salt, and pepper.
4. Stuff the mixture into the hollowed-out bell peppers.
5. Place the stuffed peppers in a baking dish and cover with foil.
6. Bake for 30-35 minutes, or until the peppers are tender.
7. If desired, remove the foil, top with grated cheese, and bake for an additional 5 minutes until the cheese is melted and bubbly.
8. Serve these quinoa and black bean stuffed peppers as a hearty appetizer.

Sweet Potato Bites with Avocado Cream

Ingredients:

- 2 sweet potatoes, sliced into rounds
- 2 tablespoons olive oil
- 1 teaspoon smoked paprika
- Salt and pepper to taste
- 1 ripe avocado
- 1/4 cup Greek yogurt
- Juice of 1 lemon
- Fresh cilantro leaves for garnish

Instructions:

1. Preheat your oven to 400°F (200°C) and line a baking sheet with parchment paper.
2. In a bowl, toss sweet potato rounds with olive oil, smoked paprika, salt, and pepper until well coated.
3. Arrange the sweet potato rounds on the baking sheet and bake for 20-25 minutes, turning once, until they are tender and slightly crispy.

4. While the sweet potatoes are baking, prepare the avocado cream. In a blender or food processor, combine the ripe avocado, Greek yogurt, lemon juice, and a pinch of salt. Blend until smooth.

5. Serve the roasted sweet potato rounds with a dollop of avocado cream and garnish with fresh cilantro leaves.

Mini Vegetable Frittatas

Ingredients:

- 6 large eggs
- 1/4 cup milk (or milk alternative)
- 1/2 cup diced bell peppers
- 1/2 cup diced zucchini
- 1/2 cup diced tomatoes
- 1/4 cup diced onions
- 1/4 cup grated cheese (optional)
- Salt and black pepper to taste
- Cooking spray or olive oil for greasing muffin tin

Instructions:

1. Preheat your oven to 350°F (175°C) and grease a muffin tin with cooking spray or olive oil.

2. In a bowl, whisk together eggs, milk, salt, and black pepper.

3. Divide the diced vegetables and grated cheese (if using) among the muffin cups.

4. Pour the egg mixture over the vegetables in each muffin cup, filling them about two-thirds full.

5. Bake for 18-20 minutes, or until the frittatas are set and lightly golden.

6. Allow them to cool slightly before serving these mini vegetable frittatas as a delightful appetizer.

Chapter 6: Desserts

Indulge your sweet tooth with these delightful dessert recipes. Each one is carefully crafted to satisfy your cravings while adhering to a kidney-friendly vegetarian diet. From creamy vegan cheesecake to guilt-free chocolate-covered strawberries, these desserts are a treat for your taste buds.

Berry and Banana Ice Cream

Ingredients:

- 2 ripe bananas, sliced and frozen
- 1 cup mixed berries (strawberries, blueberries, raspberries)
- 1/2 cup almond milk
- 1 tablespoon honey (optional)

Instructions:

1. Place frozen banana slices and mixed berries in a blender.
2. Add almond milk and honey (if desired).
3. Blend until smooth and creamy.

4. Serve immediately as soft-serve or freeze for a firmer texture.

Chocolate Avocado Mousse

Ingredients:

- 2 ripe avocados
- 1/4 cup unsweetened cocoa powder
- 1/4 cup honey or maple syrup
- 1 teaspoon vanilla extract
- Pinch of salt
- Fresh berries for garnish

Instructions:

1. Scoop out the flesh of avocados and place them in a food processor.
2. Add cocoa powder, honey or maple syrup, vanilla extract, and a pinch of salt.
3. Blend until smooth and creamy.
4. Spoon into serving dishes and garnish with fresh berries.
5. Refrigerate for at least 30 minutes before serving.

Vegan Rice Pudding

Ingredients:

- 1 cup Arborio rice
- 4 cups unsweetened almond milk
- 1/2 cup sugar
- 1 teaspoon vanilla extract
- 1/2 teaspoon ground cinnamon
- Raisins or chopped nuts for garnish (optional)

Instructions:

1. In a saucepan, combine rice and almond milk.
2. Bring to a simmer over medium heat, stirring frequently.
3. Reduce heat to low, cover, and cook for 20-25 minutes or until rice is tender.
4. Stir in sugar, vanilla extract, and ground cinnamon.
5. Cook for an additional 5 minutes, or until the mixture thickens.
6. Remove from heat and let it cool.
7. Garnish with raisins or chopped nuts if desired before serving.

Apple Cinnamon Crisp

Ingredients:

- 4 cups sliced apples
- 1 tablespoon lemon juice
- 1/2 cup rolled oats
- 1/4 cup whole wheat flour
- 1/4 cup brown sugar
- 1/2 teaspoon ground cinnamon
- 2 tablespoons unsalted butter or margarine

Instructions:

1. Preheat your oven to 350°F (175°C).
2. In a bowl, toss the sliced apples with lemon juice.
3. Place the apples in a baking dish.
4. In another bowl, combine rolled oats, whole wheat flour, brown sugar, and ground cinnamon.
5. Cut in the butter or margarine until the mixture resembles coarse crumbs.
6. Sprinkle the oat mixture over the apples.
7. Bake for 30-35 minutes or until the top is golden brown and the apples are tender.

8. Serve warm with a scoop of vanilla yogurt or a dollop of whipped cream.

Chia Seed Pudding with Berries

Ingredients:

- 1/4 cup chia seeds
- 1 cup unsweetened almond milk
- 1 tablespoon honey or maple syrup
- 1/2 teaspoon vanilla extract
- Fresh berries for topping

Instructions:

1. In a bowl, combine chia seeds, almond milk, honey or maple syrup, and vanilla extract.
2. Stir well and let it sit for 10 minutes.
3. Stir again, ensuring chia seeds are evenly distributed.
4. Refrigerate for at least 2 hours or overnight, stirring occasionally.
5. Serve with fresh berries on top.

Baked Pears with Cinnamon

Ingredients:

- 4 ripe pears, halved and cored
- 2 tablespoons honey
- 1 teaspoon ground cinnamon
- Chopped nuts for garnish (optional)
- Greek yogurt or ice cream for serving (optional)

Instructions:

1. Preheat your oven to 375°F (190°C).
2. Place pear halves in a baking dish.
3. Drizzle honey over the pears and sprinkle with ground cinnamon.
4. Cover the dish with foil and bake for 25-30 minutes, or until pears are tender.
5. Remove from the oven and let them cool slightly.
6. Garnish with chopped nuts if desired.
7. Serve with a dollop of Greek yogurt or a scoop of your favorite ice cream.

Vegan Chocolate Chip Cookies

Ingredients:

- 2 cups all-purpose flour
- 1 teaspoon baking powder
- 1/2 teaspoon baking soda
- 1/2 cup coconut oil, melted
- 1/2 cup maple syrup
- 1 teaspoon vanilla extract
- 1/2 cup dairy-free chocolate chips

Instructions:

1. Preheat your oven to 350°F (175°C).
2. In a bowl, whisk together flour, baking powder, and baking soda.
3. In another bowl, mix melted coconut oil, maple syrup, and vanilla extract.
4. Combine wet and dry ingredients until a dough forms.
5. Fold in dairy-free chocolate chips.
6. Drop spoonfuls of dough onto a baking sheet lined with parchment paper.
7. Flatten each cookie slightly.

8. Bake for 10-12 minutes or until the edges are golden brown.

9. Let them cool on a wire rack before enjoying.

Blueberry Oat Bars

Ingredients:

- 2 cups rolled oats
- 1 cup whole wheat flour
- 1/2 cup brown sugar
- 1/2 teaspoon baking powder
- 1/2 teaspoon salt
- 1/2 cup unsalted butter or margarine, melted
- 1 cup blueberry preserves

Instructions:

1. Preheat your oven to 350°F (175°C) and grease a baking pan.

2. In a bowl, combine rolled oats, whole wheat flour, brown sugar, baking powder, and salt.

3. Stir in the melted butter until the mixture is crumbly.

4. Press half of the mixture into the bottom of the prepared pan.

5. Spread the blueberry preserves over the crust.

6. Sprinkle the remaining oat mixture evenly over the preserves, pressing down lightly.

7. Bake for 30-35 minutes or until the top is golden brown.

8. Let it cool completely before cutting into bars.

Coconut Mango Sorbet

Ingredients:

- 2 ripe mangoes, peeled and diced
- 1 can (13.5 oz) coconut milk
- 1/4 cup honey or agave nectar
- 1 tablespoon lime juice
- Unsweetened shredded coconut for garnish (optional)

Instructions:

1. Place diced mangoes in a blender.

2. Add coconut milk, honey or agave nectar, and lime juice.

3. Blend until smooth.

4. Pour the mixture into an ice cream maker and churn according to the manufacturer's instructions.

5. Transfer the sorbet to a lidded container and freeze for a few hours or until firm.

6. Serve with a sprinkle of unsweetened shredded coconut if desired.

Chocolate Covered Strawberries

Ingredients:

- Fresh strawberries
- Dark chocolate chips or chunks
- White chocolate chips (optional)
- Chopped nuts or sprinkles for decoration (optional)

Instructions:

1. Wash and dry the strawberries thoroughly.

2. In a microwave-safe bowl, melt dark chocolate chips in 30-second intervals, stirring in between until smooth.

3. Dip each strawberry into the melted dark chocolate, letting any excess drip off.

4. Place them on a parchment-lined tray.

5. If desired, melt white chocolate chips and drizzle it over the dipped strawberries.

6. Sprinkle with chopped nuts or sprinkles while the chocolate is still soft.

7. Allow them to cool and harden before serving.

Pumpkin Pie Smoothie

Ingredients:

- 1 cup canned pumpkin puree
- 1 cup unsweetened almond milk
- 1 ripe banana
- 1/2 teaspoon ground cinnamon
- 1/4 teaspoon ground nutmeg
- 1/4 teaspoon ground ginger
- 1 tablespoon honey or maple syrup
- Ice cubes (optional)

Instructions:

1. In a blender, combine pumpkin puree, almond milk, banana, ground cinnamon, ground nutmeg, ground ginger, and honey or maple syrup.

2. Add ice cubes if you want a colder and thicker smoothie.

3. Blend until smooth and creamy.

4. Pour into a glass and sprinkle with a pinch of cinnamon for garnish.

Almond Joy Energy Bites

Ingredients:

- 1 cup rolled oats
- 1/2 cup almond butter
- 1/4 cup honey or agave nectar
- 1/4 cup shredded coconut
- 1/4 cup dark chocolate chips
- 1/4 cup chopped almonds
- 1/2 teaspoon vanilla extract
- Pinch of salt

Instructions:

1. In a bowl, combine rolled oats, almond butter, honey or agave nectar, shredded coconut, dark chocolate chips, chopped almonds, vanilla extract, and a pinch of salt.

2. Mix until all ingredients are well combined.

3. Roll the mixture into bite-sized balls and place them on a tray lined with parchment paper.

4. Refrigerate for at least 30 minutes to firm them up.

5. Enjoy as a quick and energizing snack.

Lemon Sorbet

Ingredients:

- 2 cups fresh lemon juice (about 8-10 lemons)
- 2 cups water
- 1 1/2 cups sugar
- Zest from 2 lemons

Instructions:

1. In a saucepan, combine water and sugar.

2. Heat over medium heat, stirring until the sugar is completely dissolved.

3. Remove from heat and let it cool.

4. Add fresh lemon juice and lemon zest to the sugar syrup.

5. Pour the mixture into an ice cream maker and churn according to the manufacturer's instructions.

6. Transfer the sorbet to a lidded container and freeze for a few hours until it's firm.

7. Serve with a twist of lemon zest for a refreshing dessert.

Vegan Cheesecake

Ingredients:

- 2 cups raw cashews, soaked overnight
- 1/2 cup coconut oil, melted
- 1/4 cup lemon juice
- 1/4 cup maple syrup
- 1 teaspoon vanilla extract
- 1 cup fresh berries for topping

Instructions:

1. Drain and rinse the soaked cashews.

2. In a food processor or blender, combine cashews, melted coconut oil, lemon juice, maple syrup, and vanilla extract.

3. Blend until smooth and creamy.

4. Pour the mixture into a lined cake pan and smooth the top.

5. Refrigerate for at least 4 hours or until set.

6. Top with fresh berries before serving.

Mixed Berry Parfait

Ingredients:

- 1 cup mixed berries (strawberries, blueberries, raspberries)
- 1 cup Greek yogurt or dairy-free yogurt
- 1/2 cup granola
- Honey or maple syrup for drizzling (optional)

Instructions:

1. In a glass or bowl, layer 1/4 cup of yogurt.

2. Add a layer of mixed berries.

3. Sprinkle with granola.

4. Repeat the layers.

5. Drizzle with honey or maple syrup if desired.

6. Serve immediately for a delightful parfait.

Carrot Cake Muffins

Ingredients:

- 1 1/2 cups grated carrots
- 1/2 cup unsweetened applesauce
- 1/2 cup maple syrup
- 1/4 cup vegetable oil
- 1 teaspoon vanilla extract
- 1 1/2 cups whole wheat flour
- 1/2 teaspoon baking powder
- 1/2 teaspoon baking soda
- 1/2 teaspoon ground cinnamon
- 1/4 teaspoon ground nutmeg
- 1/4 teaspoon salt
- Chopped walnuts or raisins (optional)

Instructions:

1. Preheat your oven to 350°F (175°C) and line a muffin tin with paper liners.
2. In a bowl, combine grated carrots, applesauce, maple syrup, vegetable oil, and vanilla extract.

3. In another bowl, whisk together whole wheat flour, baking powder, baking soda, ground cinnamon, ground nutmeg, and salt.

4. Combine the wet and dry ingredients, mixing until just combined.

5. Fold in chopped walnuts or raisins if desired.

6. Divide the batter into muffin cups.

7. Bake for 20-25 minutes or until a toothpick comes out clean when inserted into a muffin.

8. Let them cool before enjoying.

Chocolate Zucchini Bread

Ingredients:

- 1 1/2 cups grated zucchini
- 1/2 cup unsweetened cocoa powder
- 1 1/2 cups whole wheat flour
- 1/2 cup brown sugar
- 1/4 cup vegetable oil
- 2 eggs (or egg substitute for vegans)
- 1 teaspoon vanilla extract
- 1/2 teaspoon baking soda
- 1/2 teaspoon baking powder

- 1/2 teaspoon salt
- 1/2 cup dairy-free chocolate chips (optional)

Instructions:

1. Preheat your oven to 350°F (175°C) and grease a loaf pan.
2. In a bowl, combine grated zucchini and cocoa powder.
3. In another bowl, mix whole wheat flour, brown sugar, vegetable oil, eggs or egg substitute, vanilla extract, baking soda, baking powder, and salt.
4. Combine the zucchini mixture with the flour mixture and stir until well combined.
5. Fold in dairy-free chocolate chips if desired.
6. Pour the batter into the prepared loaf pan.
7. Bake for 50-60 minutes or until a toothpick comes out clean when inserted into the center.
8. Let it cool before slicing.

Peanut Butter Banana Ice Cream

Ingredients:

- 4 ripe bananas, sliced and frozen

- 2 tablespoons peanut butter
- 2 tablespoons cocoa powder (optional)
- Chopped peanuts for garnish (optional)

Instructions:

1. Place frozen banana slices in a blender.
2. Add peanut butter and cocoa powder if desired.
3. Blend until smooth and creamy.
4. Serve immediately with a sprinkle of chopped peanuts if desired.

CONCLUSION

As we embark on a journey of reflection and empowerment. Your exploration of vegetarian kidney-friendly cuisine has reached its final destination, but it's only the beginning of your personal wellness voyage. Let's take a moment to recap the incredible flavors, nourishment, and care that you've experienced throughout this cookbook.

As you close the pages of this cookbook, remember that your commitment to a kidney-conscious vegetarian diet is a lifelong investment in your health. It's not just about recipes; it's about making mindful choices every day. It's about savoring the vibrant colors and tastes of fresh ingredients while protecting your kidneys.

We hope this cookbook has not only provided you with delicious recipes but also inspired you to get creative in your kitchen. Don't be afraid to tweak recipes to suit your taste and dietary needs. Cooking is an art, and you are the artist. Embrace the joy of experimenting with flavors, textures, and ingredients.

Maintaining a kidney-friendly diet can be challenging at times, but remember that you're not alone on this journey. Seek support from your healthcare provider, join online communities, or share your experiences with friends and family. Together, we can make kidney health a priority and savor the joys of delicious, nourishing food.

In this concluding chapter, we'd like to express our gratitude for choosing this cookbook as your guide. We sincerely hope it has enriched your culinary repertoire and, more importantly, improved your well-being. As you continue your path to health and vitality, may your kitchen always be filled with love, laughter, and the delightful aromas of kidney-friendly vegetarian cuisine.

Thank you for allowing us to be part of your journey to better kidney health. Wishing you a lifetime of good health and countless delicious meals.